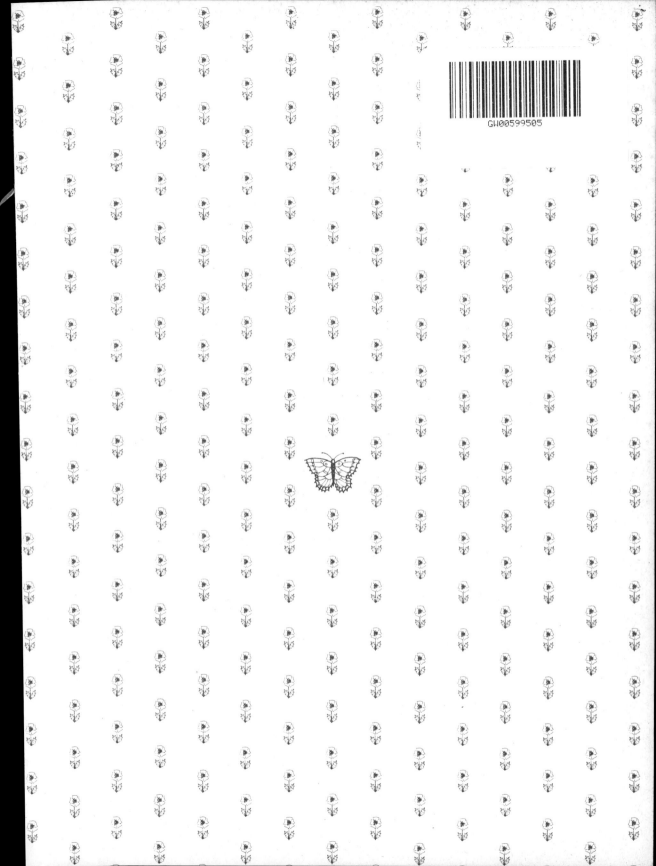

GW00599505

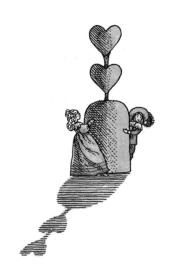

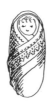

First published in Great Britain 1985 by
Webb & Bower (Publishers) Limited
9 Colleton Crescent, Exeter, Devon EX2 4BY

Illustration and Design Sue Warne

Production Nick Facer

British Library Cataloguing in Publication Data

Culpeper, Nicholas
Culpeper's book of birth.
1. Pregnancy   2. Childbirth
I. Title   II. Thomas, Ian
618.2   RG524
ISBN 0-86350-041-2

Typeset in Great Britain by P&M Typesetting Ltd.,
Exeter, Devon

Printed and bound in Italy by
New Interlitho SpA

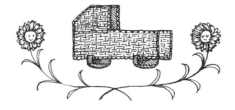

CULPEPER'S BOOK of BIRTH

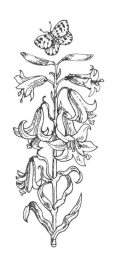

Edited and with an Introduction
by Ian Thomas
Illustrated by Sue Warne
Foreword by Mrs. Betty Parsons

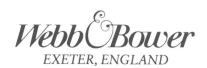

Webb & Bower
EXETER, ENGLAND

Foreword

I feel honoured to have been asked to write the Foreword to this book, knowing that all the royalties from its sale will go to Birthright, the Charity of the Royal College of Obstetricians and Gynaecologists, which is doing such remarkable work in helping to make pregnancy and childbirth safer for mothers and babies.

Nicholas Culpeper recorded his research over three hundred years ago. Much has changed in the obstetrical and pediatric field since then, for which we can be grateful. The hazards of pregnancy and childbirth which threatened the safety of mother and baby then, have to a great extent been eliminated by advances in medical science and modern technology. Much has still to be done, but great steps forward have been taken.

But many basic ideas remain the same: the need for a good diet, moderate exercise, rest and relaxation. It seems from reading Nicholas Culpeper's observations that women's emotions have not changed very much. They will have the same fears and hopes that their sisters had three hundred years ago. It is interesting too that then, as now, women took dislikes to certain food during pregnancy, and developed desires for others. In all my experience I have never heard of anyone with a craving for coals or ashes, but did they perhaps have an instinctive need for calcium, minerals and other such elements?

Many of the seventeenth-century ideas must be adjusted to the twentieth century. We know that it is not wise to keep a woman lying still for a week after delivery. Static nursing can cause thrombosis. Mothers and babies are allowed to be bathed more often than was the case in the seventeenth century. Fathers play a role today which would have been unthinkable three hundred years ago. The scientific advantages of today, in a post-Pasteur situation safeguard against infections which caused so much infant and maternal mortality.

But there is wisdom underlying much of what Culpeper writes about which is eternal: for instance the relationship between a happy, contented, unfatigued mother and her child. We can learn so much from the past. If we can balance this wisdom with the scientific knowledge of today, we will be able to make pregnancy, childbirth and parenthood both physically safer and emotionally more satisfying for all concerned.

I have enjoyed this book. It is easy to read. It is amusing and thought-provoking. I am sure it will bring pleasure and interest to anyone who reads it.

Betty Parsons

Mrs. Betty Parsons is a trained nurse. She has taught relaxation for 30 years to over 17,000 women.

A Seventeenth Century Guide to Having Lusty Children

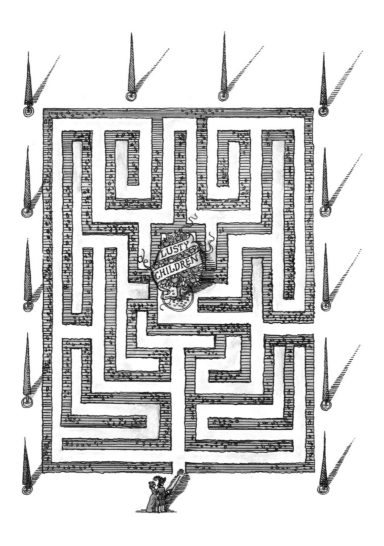

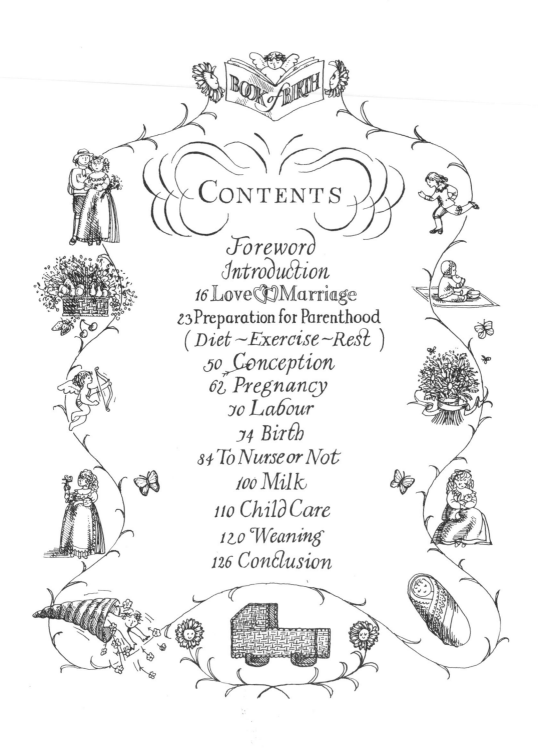

CONTENTS

BOOK of BIRTH

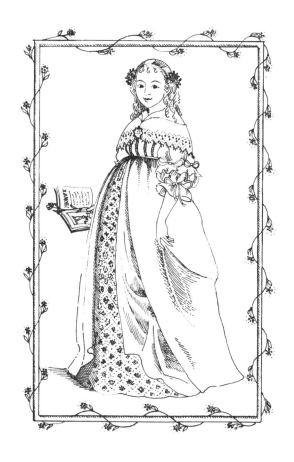

I desire that my book should be
for everyone's good and therefore
within the reach of everyone's purse,
and rest confident. There is enough in it
to employ the brains of the wisest woman
breathing, and to do the silliest good

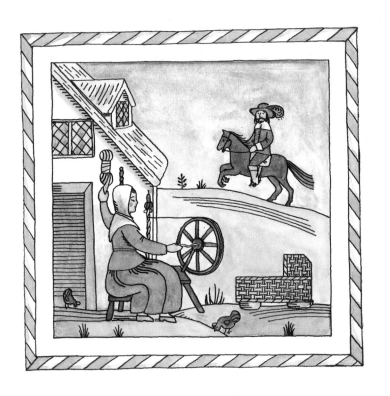

INTRODUCTION BY IAN THOMAS

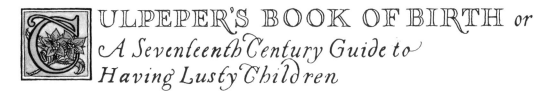

CULPEPER'S BOOK OF BIRTH *or* A Seventeenth Century Guide to Having Lusty Children

These extracts are taken from Nicholas Culpeper's
A Directory for Midwives published over 300 years ago.
They give an insight into what life was like for the mother
of seventeenth century England; certainly not as Merrie
as sometimes made out. Disease was endemic, water
contaminated, hygiene non-existent, washing rare,
sanitary habits 'free and filthy', infant
mortality levels seen today only in the most
primitive parts of the world.

     Against this background,
Culpeper's advice to his women readers is
remarkable: clear, well expressed, tender
of mother and child, sensitive and at times,
very funny.

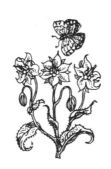

" They being most fit for English bodies."

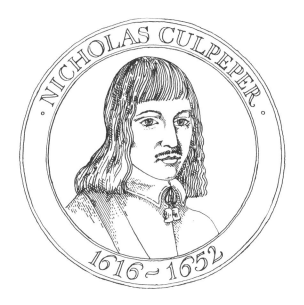

icholas Culpeper (1616-1652) is the best
known of the famous English herbalists. He
was the first person to translate the
Pharmacopaea of the London College of
Physicians from Latin into English. Hitherto secret
doctors' knowledge was thus made available to the
ordinary person in his own language. He was the first
person to produce a truly English herbal, one based on
plants that could be found in any English garden, 'they
being most fit for English bodies'. Since herbal
medicines were the only medicines, and herbs from
one's own garden cost next to nothing, the book was an
immediate success. It is this book, *The English
Physician*, published continuously since as the *Culpeper
Herbal* , for which he is best known today.

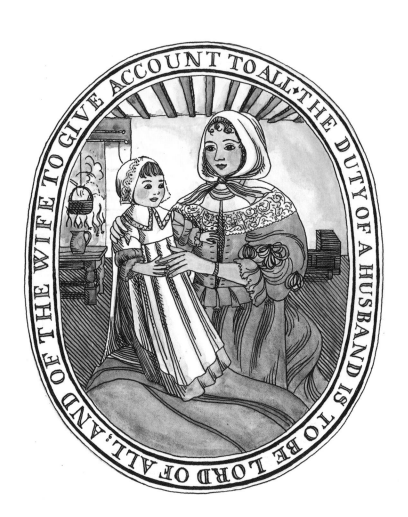

THE DUTY OF A HUSBAND IS TO BE LORD OF ALL; AND OF THE WIFE TO GIVE ACCOUNT TO ALL. THE

Directory for Midwives was published in 1651. The Directory, its secondary title *A Guide for Women in Their Conception, Bearing and Suckling their Children*, was reprinted at least seventeen times, the last time in 1777. It was Culpeper's most popular book after *The English Physician*.

There was good reason for its popularity. Until the Industrial Revolution of the nineteenth century, the bulk of the population lived outside the towns. Only in the towns were there doctors, these few in number. So it was the women at home who made their traditional lotions and potions; who cared and looked after the sick, and who helped bring forth the babies. In the seventeenth century, 'the duty of a husband is to be Lord of all; and of the wife to give account of all'. Any book that could help women in one of their prime tasks was bound to be of interest, particularly one written by the now celebrated Nicholas Culpeper, 'Gent. Student in Physick and Astrology'.

Culpeper's interest in women and their children was a real one. It was touched by his own experiences: 'myself having buried many of my children young caused me to fix my thoughts intently on this business'. His was a sadness of the times. Of his seven children only one survived infancy.

f he wrote from personal experience, he also wrote with authority and considerable humour. Then as now the controversy raged as to whether you should feed your own child or not. 'Oh! what a raket do authors make about this, what thwarting and contradicting'. If you did not feed your child yourself, you needed a nurse. A nurse in the seventeenth century was not a well educated girl trained to look after children, but a woman who had lost her own baby and still had her own milk. She was a wet-nurse. There were plenty to hand. About one-fifth of all children died in infancy. Your wet nurse was thus available to feed your child if you were unable to do so yourself, or if it was felt it was unwise . . . or if as happens today, the mother's feeding did not fit in with the routine around the baby! The most common reason was, however, the desire or need of the mother to become pregnant again. If she was feeding her own baby, this was not possible.

Like the modern au-pair, it was important that the nurse fitted in to the family. There were all sorts of ways that you could tell whether you had chosen a good nurse or not. Her character, humours, eating and drinking habits all had to be taken into account. Even your baby was to be considered. You were advised to choose a nurse with 'good nipples so that the child will take to them with pleasure'.

he language is of the time: very direct. As Culpeper put it, he did not want to offend his women readers (since his intention was to please them in his treatise, if doing them good will please them) but he was not going to 'muffle up their eyes' to prevent them seeing the truth. 'I want fit English terms to express them, unless I would coin them, and that I leave to be done by such as effect novelties'. So his advice is expressed in good earthy English and very clear it is.

Culpeper seems very modern in his attitude to sensible diet and exercise. He recognized also the importance of clean fresh air. But not the importance of clean water. It seems so obvious today looking back. No doubt the people in later years will look at us in equal astonishment wondering why on earth we could not see the damage we were doing our bodies with junk food, excessive tranquilisers and sleeping pills, medicines that are more concerned with profitable instant relief than simple prevention.

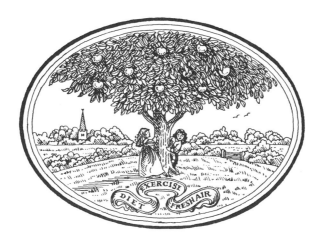

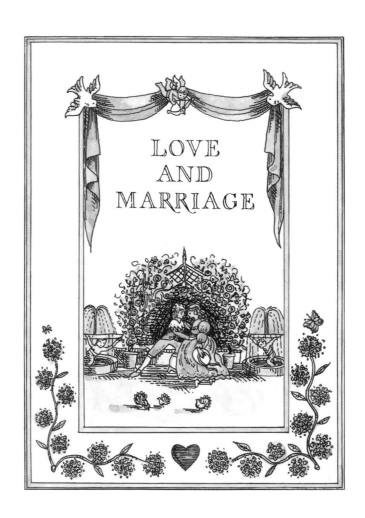

LOVE
AND
MARRIAGE

Marriage is the greatest natural action of man's life, and he that waits upon God for his direction of it shall not do so amiss.

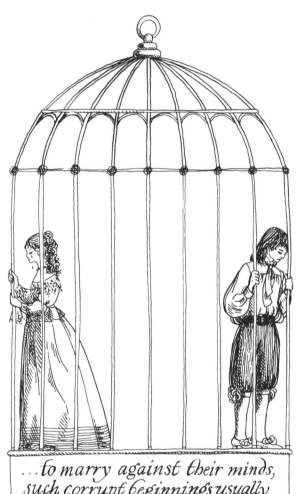

...to marry against their minds,
such corrupt beginnings usually
bring forth sorrow enough to all parties

It is a sad thing that men did take women from their friends that did love them, and then hate them; and as sad as women when they are married should either through pride or folly, or something else, so forget themselves, their husbands and their God, that they cannot live quietly with them, and worse than either (if worse can be) is that trick of parents to compel their children to marry against their minds, such corrupt beginnings usually bring forth sorrow enough to all parties.

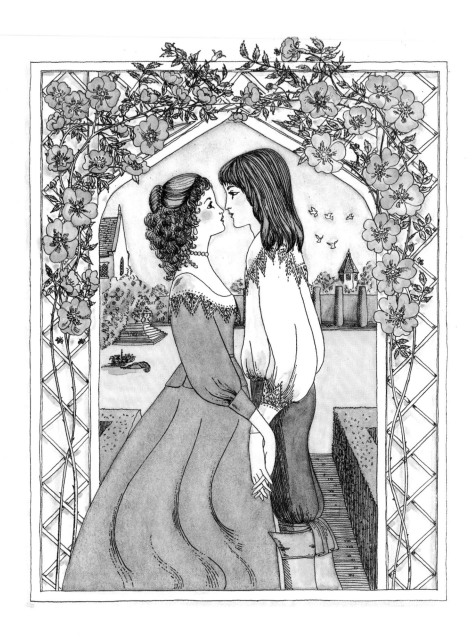

Men and women beget men and women, then if their hearts be not united in love, how should their seed unite to cause conception?

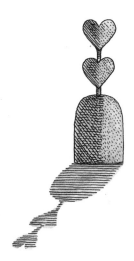

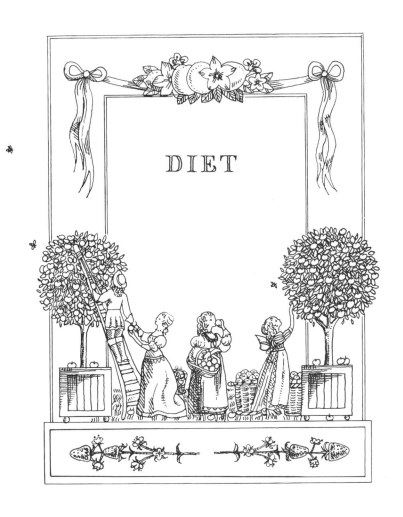

DIET

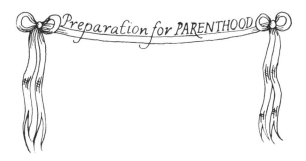

Preparation for PARENTHOOD

I shall be very brief in laying down this . . . and not tire your patience with the tale of a cock and a bull; therefore consider that by a temperate diet I intend that such an exact quantity of meat and drink should be taken into the stomach, as the stomach is well able to concoct and digest perfectly which sufficeth the due nourishment of the body.

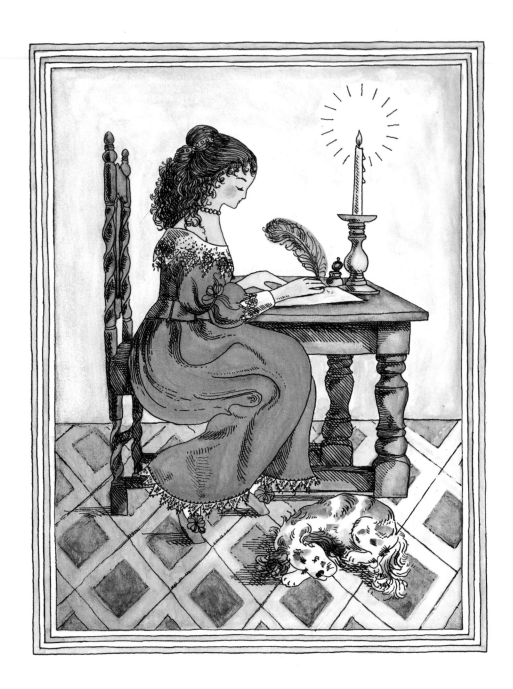

That such as lead a studious life ought not to eat as much as those that lead a laborious life, because the digestion is not so good, therefore their meats ought to be less in quantity and lighter in digestion.

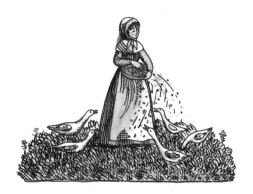

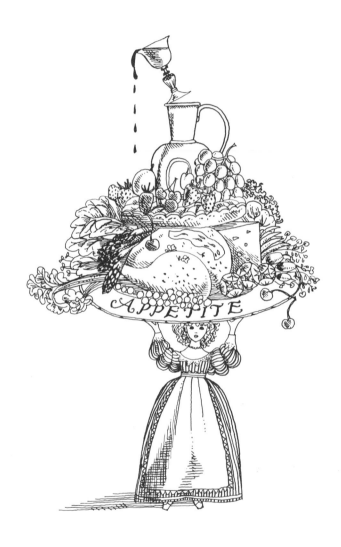

Appetite is many times prolonged beyond the satisfaction of hunger or thirst, so that three or four times of such as would suffice nature is thrust into the body of liquorishness.

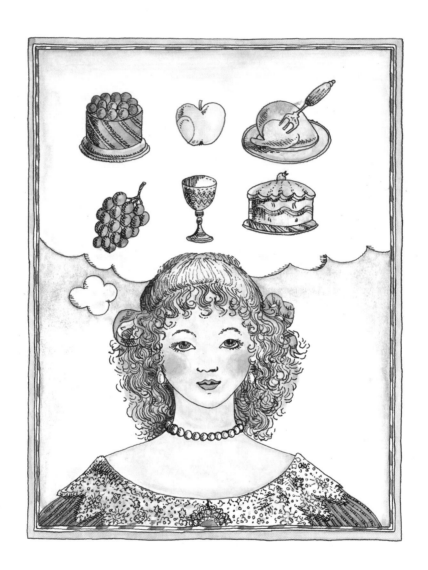

Appetite many times preceeds from the apprehension of the fancy; fancy conceives meats to be delightful and pleasant, and appetite follows that, when reason itself testifies it to be hurtful.

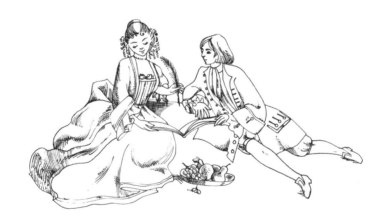

If you take so much food at a time as makes you unfit for study and other duties of the mind, then it is apparent you have exceeded the due measure; for it is very clear that all the offence that proceeds to the brain by way of food arises from the abundance of vapours which are sent up from the stomach to the head which either would not be at all, or else would be pure if you had not eat and drunk too much.

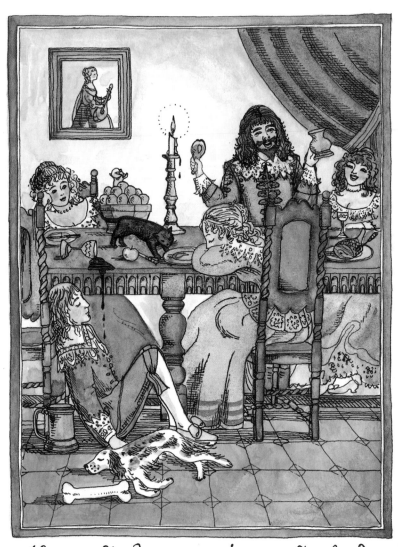

If you find a weariness after food,
be sure you have taken too much.

If you find a dullness, heaviness and weariness after food, or a proneness so soon as you have eaten, be sure you have taken too much; for meat and drink ought to refresh the body and make it cheerful, and not oppress it and make it dull.

Subtract from your excess in diet by little by little for *"Nature abhors all sudden changes, though they be from bad to good"*; as ill custome got possession over nature by degrees, so let it be outed by degrees.

When the stomach receives more food than it can digest, the chyle made of such meat must needs be crude, because the stomach maketh a corruption instead of a concoction.

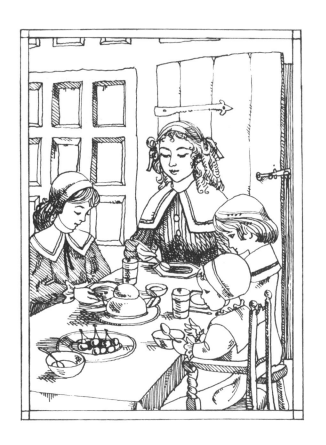

From a temperate diet is good chyle caused. Such as is agreeable to nature, from good chyle is good blood bred, and from good blood good seed, and from good seed, strong children, lusty and healthful which according to the principles of nature are subject to live.

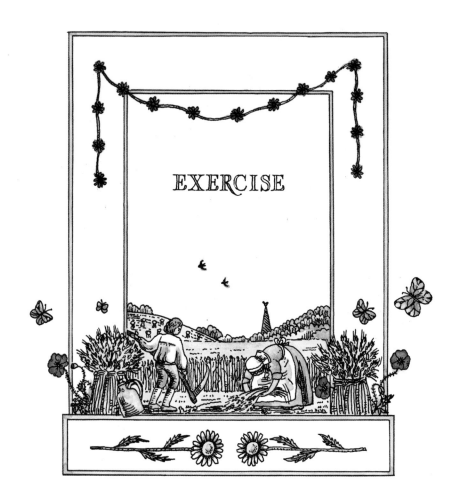

EXERCISE

That ever God ordained men and women to live idly, I never yet read or heard; and Lycurgus, that famous Spartan commander, being asked the reason why he forced young virgins to labour, answered very wisely and discreetly, that thereby cleansing their bodies of evil excrements, they might bring forward lusty children when they were married.

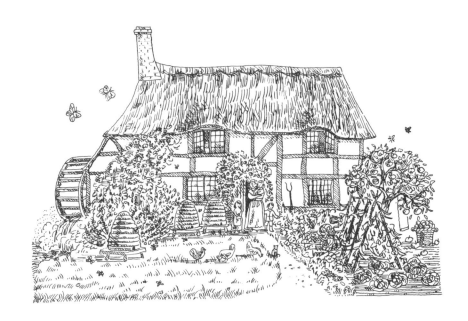

That poor people such as work hard, and fare hard, and are seldom idle, have more children, and those stronger and lustier of body, and usually longer lived than those that live idly and fare deliciously.

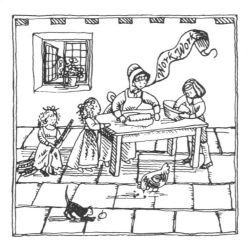

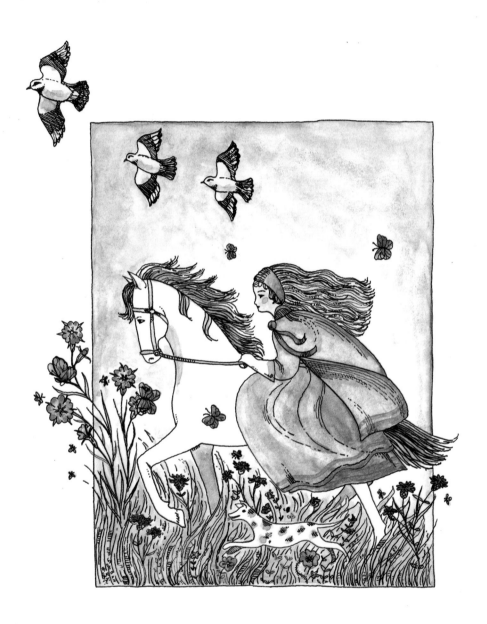

How the exercise of the body of the parent conduceth to the life of the child . . . it stirs up natural heat in them. There is much difference between a man's body when natural heat is stirred up, and when it is not stirred up, as there is between the earth in winter and summer. When the sun stirs up natural heat in the elements, the earth rejoyceth and brings forth its increase. When the sun departs and by its distance cannot stir up natural heat, then the earth is dismantled of the beauty bestoweth upon her and mourns like the trees in October.

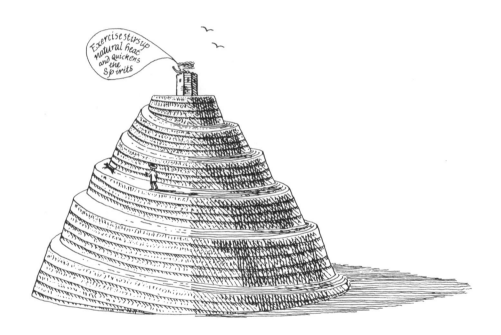

Even so in the body of man, if natural heat be stirred up by moderate exercise, it will be active and capable of concocting pure and good seed for the generation of man.

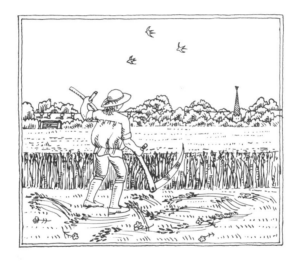

Moderate exercise equally distributes the spirits throughout the body, and if so, then of necessity they must needs be distributed equally in the seed.

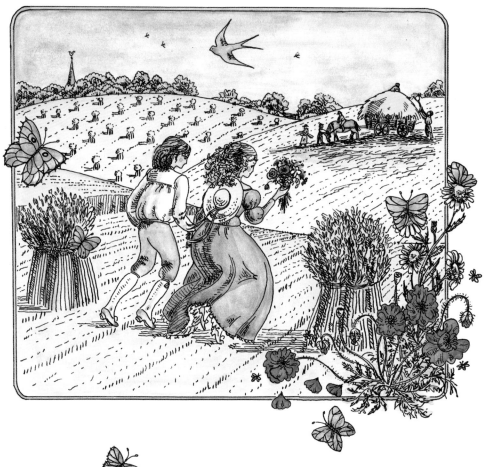

Moderate exercise by opening the pores, cleaneth the blood of those fuliginous and sooty vapours which usually offend it; and this is the reason sweating is such a good remedy in feavours. Now then, if the blood be cleansed of what offends it, or corrupts it before it be sent down to the testicles to be conducted into seed, the children bred of this purified seed must needs be stronger and by consequence more subject to live. Moderate exercise of the parents conduceth much to the lives of the children.

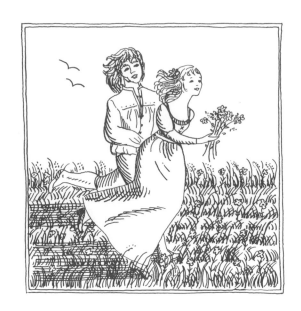

Moderate Exercise

1 Stirs up natural heat.
2 Quickens the spirits.
3 Opens the pores.
4 Wasts the excrements of the third digestion.
5 Makes the body, senses and spirits strong, and
  that's the way to have strong children.
6 Comforts all the limbs.
7 Helps nature in all her exercises, of which
  procreation of children is not the least.

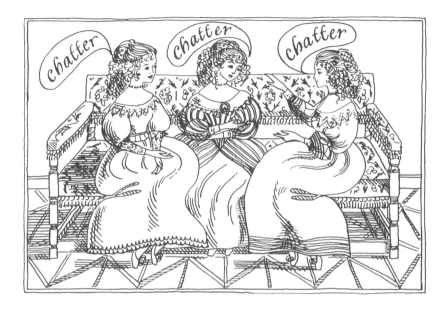

Immoderate Exercise (which is a thing our
city dames are utterly unaquainted with, unless it be
the exercise of their tongues)

1 Wastes, dries, consumes, wearies both bodies and
   spirits.
2 Hurts the body in every part.
3 Overthrows nature's actions.

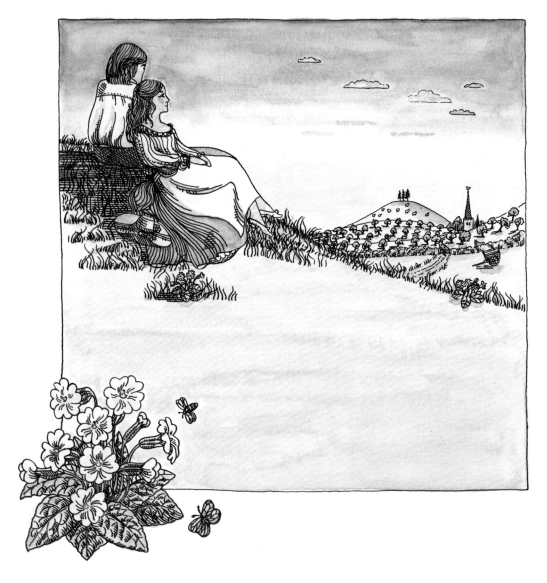

Moderate Rest

1 Comforteth and refresheth nature.
2 Recruits a tired brain.
3 Maintains health.
4 Strengthens both body, senses and members.

Immoderate Rest

1 Dulls both mind, senses and principal
   instruments of the body.
2 Causeth . . . half the infirmities that accompany
   the body of man and woman.
3 It hastens old age.
4 It causeth deformity: hark you women, if you
   would be young and fair, use yourselves to labor.

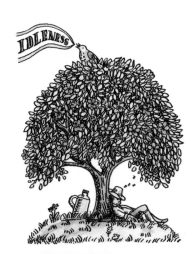

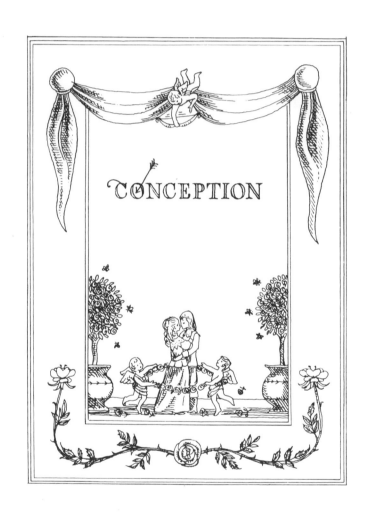

CONCEPTION

The instruments of generation are of two sorts, male and female: their use is the procreation of mankind; their operation is by action and passion, the agent is the seed, the patient blood; so that the body of man being composed by action and passion, he must needs during his life, be subject to them both.

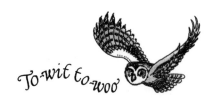

To-wit to-woo

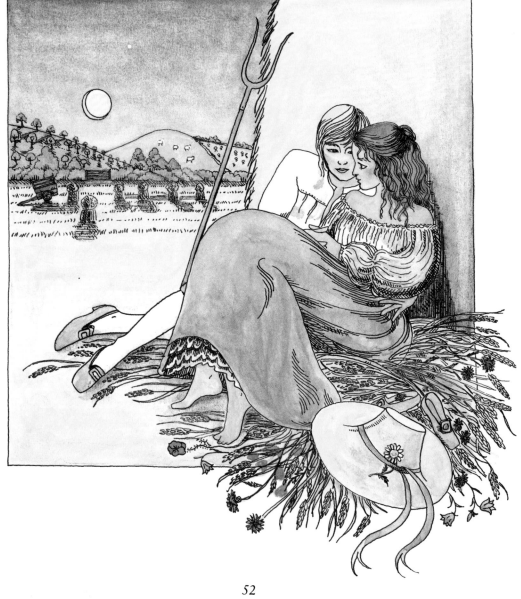

It is most certain, that all men and women desire children partly because they are blessings of God . . . or else because they are pretty things to play withal, every like desiring to play with his like, or lastly, and most probably, lust is the cause of begetting more children than the desire of the blessings of God, for where the desire of children moves one to the act of copulation, the pleasure in the act moves an hundred.

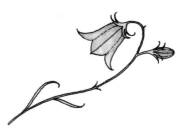

In the act of copulation, the woman spends her
seed as well as the man, and both are united to
make the conception.

The seeds of both sexes being united, the
womb instantly shuts up, partly to hinder the
extramission or passing out of the seed, partly to
cherish the seed by its inbred heat, the better to
provoke it to action . . . then instantly nature goes
to work.

The first thing which is operative in the
conception is the spirit, whereof the seed is full.

The reason why a male is conceived, sometimes a
female, is the strength of the seed. If the man's
seed be strongest, a male is conceived; if the
woman's, a female. The greater light obscures the
lesser, by the same rule and that's the reason why
weakly men get most girls, if they get any children at
all. There shews a manifest difference between
nature and appetite: nature strives to beget its like.
Men to beget men, women to beget women: but the
men desire girls, and women boys, is appetite
not nature.

Use not the act of copulation too often . . . Satiety
gluts the womb, and makes it unfit to do its
offices and that's the reason whores have so seldome
children, and also the reason why women after long
absence of their husbands, when they come again,
usually soon conceive.

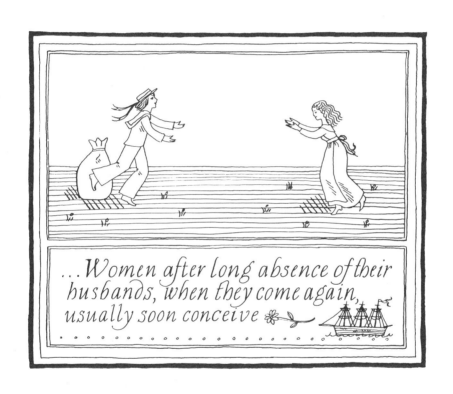

...Women after long absence of their husbands, when they come again, usually soon conceive

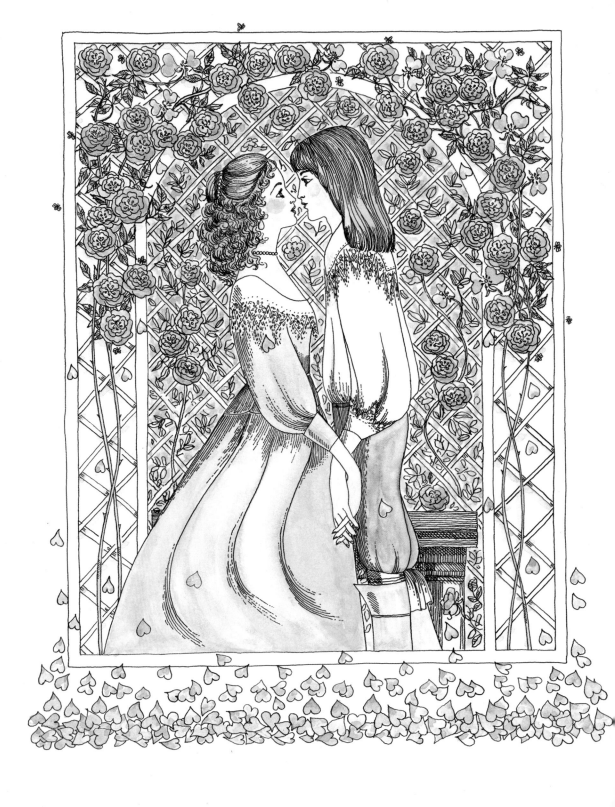

Let the time be convenient, for fear of surprise hinders conception. Let it be after perfect digestion. Let neither hunger nor drunkenness be upon the man or woman.

Exercise your body before you take counsel of the under sheet. Go to the school of Mars before you go to the school of Venus.

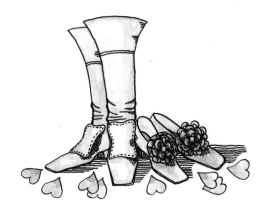

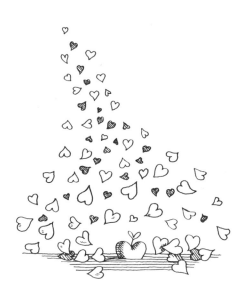

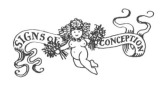

If she keeps the seed, it is a sign she hath conceived, and a man may know that the seed is kept, if he find in copulation that his yard is sucked and drawn by the womb, and the privities are not moist.

The chiefest sign of conception is, when there is at first loathing of meat, pewking pica, or preter natural appetite and vomiting. And when they hate that they earnestly affected, or faint when they think of them.

And this is when the child takes the purest blood, and leaves the impure, which gets into the mouth of the stomach and infects it, and hence comes the loathing of some sorts of meats.
Pica is when they desire strange and absurd things as coals, ashes etc.

Signs of conception:
Tops of the nipples look redder than normally
. . . The breasts begin to swell and wax hard, not without pain and soreness. The veins of the breasts are more clearly seen than they were wont to be.

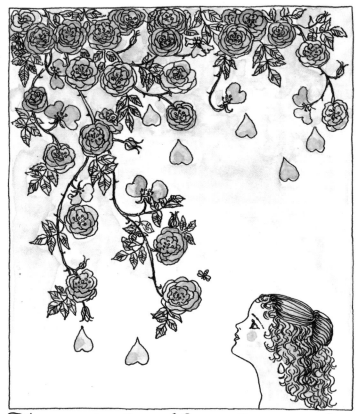

The imagination of the mother operates
most forcibly in the conception of the
child. How much better then were it
for women to lead contented lives, that so
their imaginations may be pure and clear,
that so that their conception may be well formed.

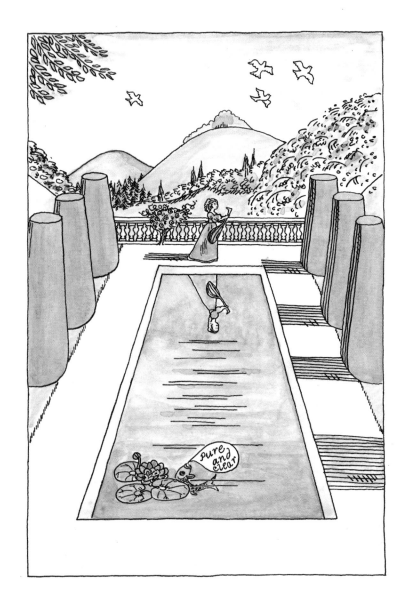

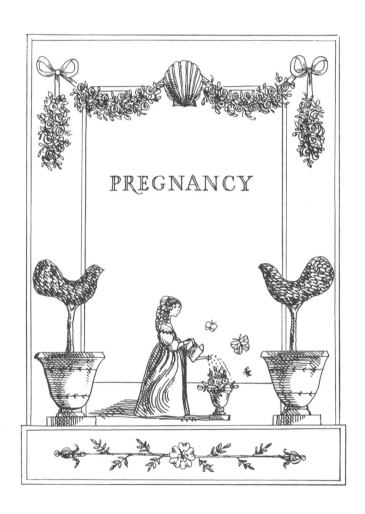

PREGNANCY

Your child is nourished by your own blood, your blood is bred by your own diet rectified or marred by your exercise, idleness, sleep or watching etc. Nature sees and knows how you swerved from what is fitting.

Discontent stirs up such affections in the body as are inimical both to body and mind and therefore must needs . . . spoil the child in the womb; such are anger, passion, hatred, fear of things to come, fear for things past, sorrow, sighing and grief of mind. All these corrupt the very nourishment wherewith the child is nourished in the womb, and often times kills the fruit in its very bud.

What a foolish thing it is to do yourselves so great a mischief, with not the least hope of doing yourselves the least good.

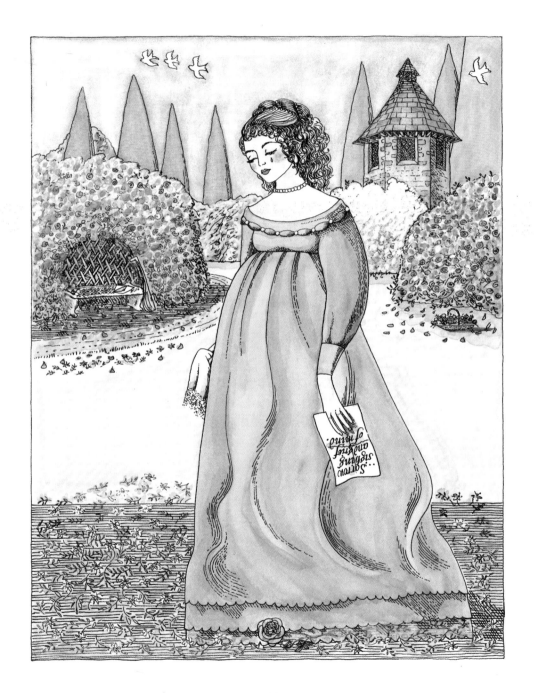

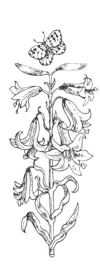

Of the government and diet of woman with child. Let meate be easy of concoction; let her eat quinces to strengthen the child, or sweet almonds with honey, sweet apples, grapes. Let her abstain from sharp meats, very bitter or salt, and things that can provoke terms, as garlick, onions, olives, mustard, fennel, pepper, and all spices. In the last months cinnamon is good. Summer fruits are naught for her, and all pulse. When the child is bigger, let her diet be more, for it is better for women with child to eat too much than too little, lest the child want nourishment.

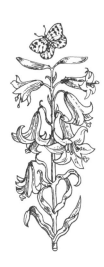

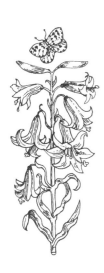

Let her drink moderately of clear wine, not exercise too much, nor dance, nor ride in a coach that shakes her; let her not lift any great weights in the first and last months. In the ninth month, let her move a little more, to dilate the parts and stir up natural heat. After the fourth month, women prevent wrinkles by carrying a clout upon the belly, dipt in oyl of sweet almonds, jesamine, oyl of lillies to loosen the skin, that it may stretch better without clefts.

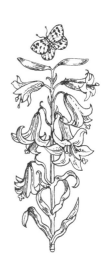

She may bathe in the last months, once in
a week to loosen the privy parts. Let her
avoid anger, sorrow, fear and too much mirth.
Let her sleep rather than be watchful.
Let the belly be kept loose in the first month, with
prunes, raisins, or manna in broth.

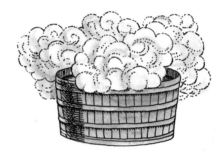

When the child can no longer be contained in so
small a place, being grown and requiring
more nourishment, it kicks and breaks the
membranes and ligaments that held it, and the
womb by expelling faculty, sends it forth with great
straining, and this is called travel. The child comes
with the head forward and the heels upwards, with
his hands and arms to his thighs, and so the other
parts easily follow . . . it seems to fall rather than be
expelled, and the bones of the privities must needs
be divided.

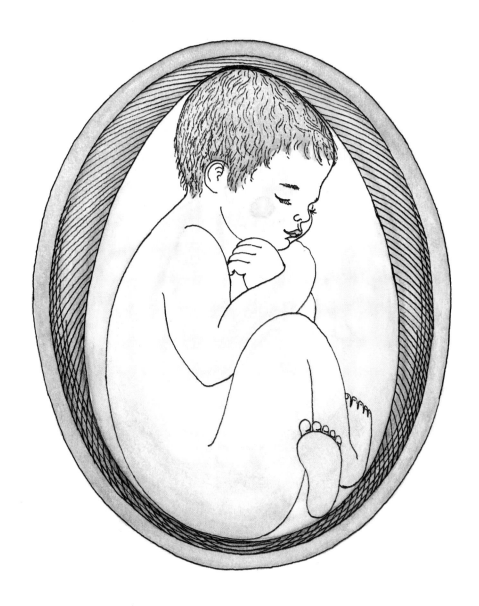

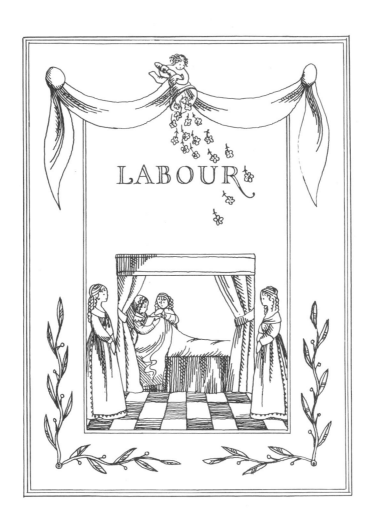

LABOUR

Though child-bearing since Eve's sin is ordained to be painful as a punishment thereof, yet sometimes it is more painful than ordinary.

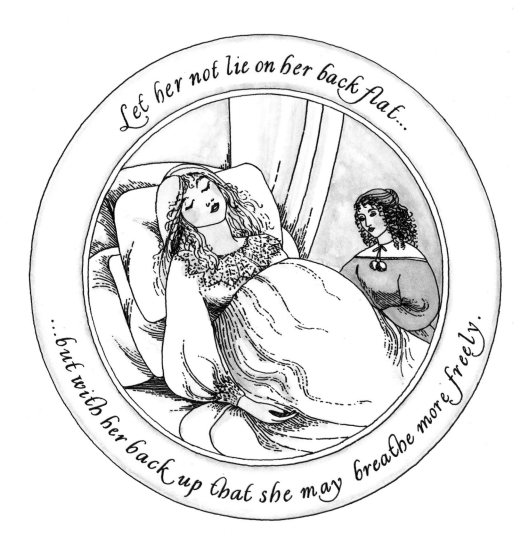

Let her not lie on her back flat... ...but with her back up that she may breathe more freely.

L et her not lie on her back flat but with her back up
that she may breathe more freely.

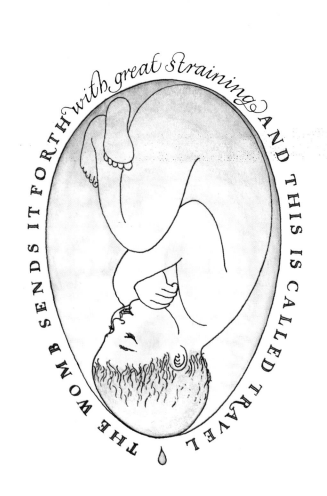

THE WOMB SENDS IT FORTH *with great straining* AND THIS IS CALLED TRAVEL

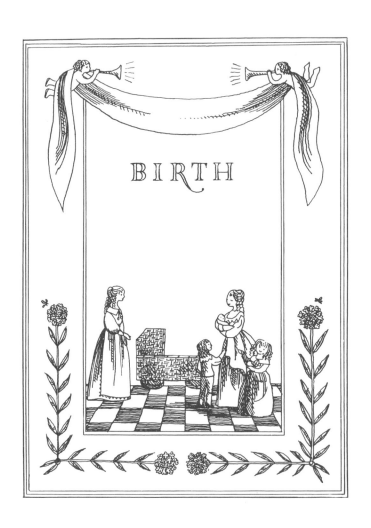

BIRTH

If her body be exceeding weak, keep her not too hot. Extremity of heat wakens nature and dissolves the strength.

Secondly, be she weak or strong, let no cold come near her at first.

Thirdly, let her diet be hot and let her eat but little at a time. Let her the first three daies (and longer if she be weak) avoid the light. Her labour weakens her eyes exceedingly by a harmony between the womb and them. Let her avoid great noises and sadness, together with trouble of mind; for whether it should be most fitting she should be praising God for her delivery, or troubled about the wagging of a straw, judge you.

Compose her in bed, and give her good food. Let the air be temperate, rather hot than cold.

If travel be hard, anoint the belly and sides with oyl of sweet almonds, lillies and sweet wine.

Let her meat be of good juyce and easie concoction, hen broth, and chickens and capons, kid, mutton, veal.

Let her drink thin wine if there be no feaver, or cinnamon boyled in water, the first daies drunk warm, and let her not rise too soon.

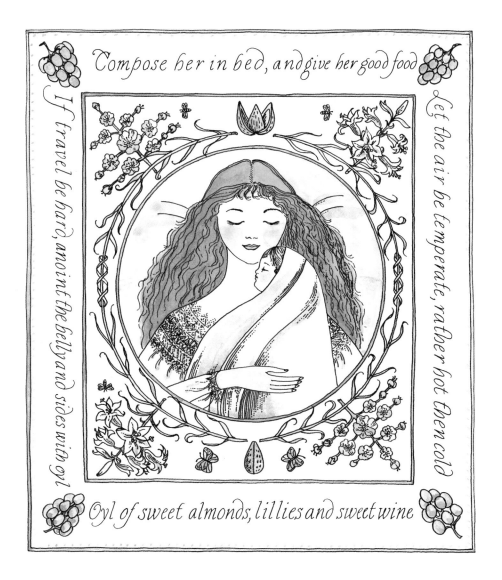

Compose her in bed, and give her good food

Let the air be temperate, rather hot then cold

If travel be hard, anoint the belly and sides with oyl

Oyl of sweet almonds, lillies and sweet wine

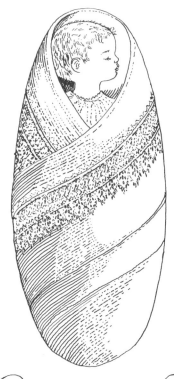

Let her avoid
trouble of the mind...
It should be most fitting
she should be praising God
for her delivery

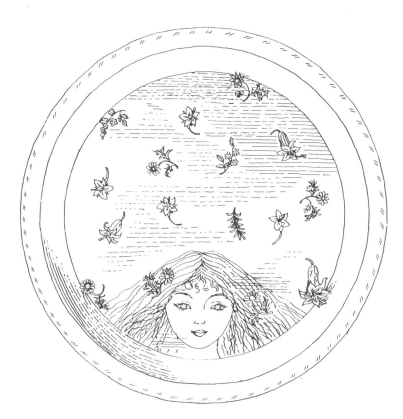

Before she goes forth, let her bath with a
decoction of lilly roots, elicampane, mugwort,
agrimony, borage, rosemary, chamomil flowers,
staechas, fenugreek, linseed and citron peels.

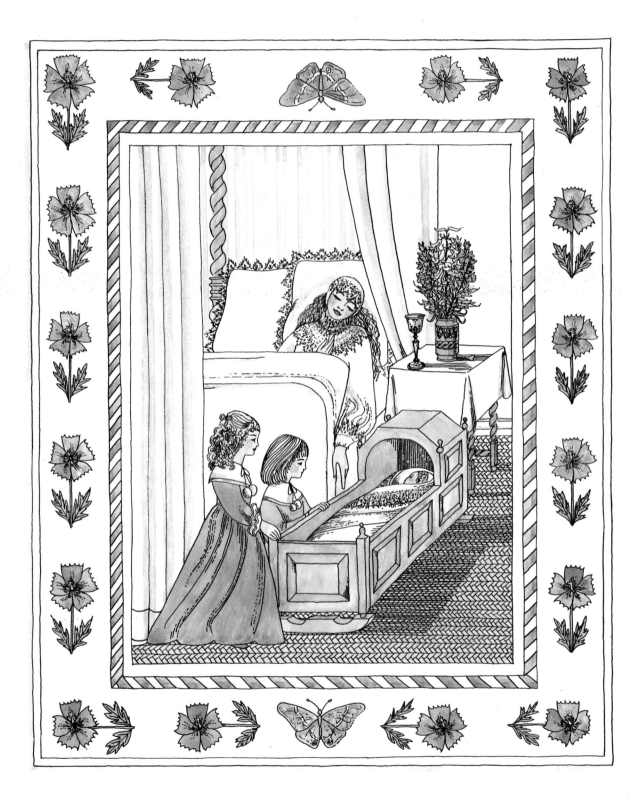

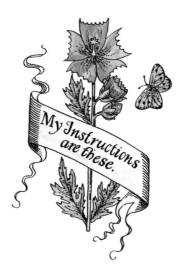

My instructions are these.
So soon as she is laid in her bed, let her drink a draught of burnt white wine, in which you have melted a dram of spermaceti.

Let her stir as little as maybe till after the fifth, sixth and seventh daies after delivery, if she be weak. Let her talk as little as may be, for it weakens her. Gossips tales do women little good in such a case.
If she goes not well to stool, give her a clyster, made only with the decoction of mallows, and a little red sugar.

Gather Vervain in May and June

When she hath lyen in a week, or something more, let her use such things as close the womb: of which knotgrass and comfry bear away the bell; you may if you please add a little purging to it and do yourselves no harm; put in both polypodium both leaves and roots bruised. Our Colledg of Physitians, and so do the ancients also affirm, that polypodium of the oak is to be preferred before all other polypodiums whatsoever. I know of no other reason they have for it, but only because it is more scarce, and because more scarce, more dear, and because more dear, it brings more money, and that's the grease makes the wheels go.

OAK?

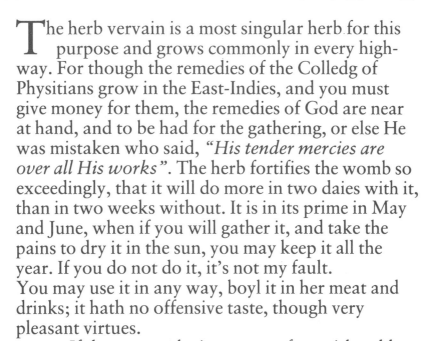

The herb vervain is a most singular herb for this purpose and grows commonly in every highway. For though the remedies of the Colledg of Physitians grow in the East-Indies, and you must give money for them, the remedies of God are near at hand, and to be had for the gathering, or else He was mistaken who said, *"His tender mercies are over all His works"*. The herb fortifies the womb so exceedingly, that it will do more in two daies with it, than in two weeks without. It is in its prime in May and June, when if you will gather it, and take the pains to dry it in the sun, you may keep it all the year. If you do not do it, it's not my fault.
You may use it in any way, boyl it in her meat and drinks; it hath no offensive taste, though very pleasant virtues.

If the woman be in any way feaverish, add plantane to it, whether leaves or roots, it matters not. If she be not feaverish, it will not do amiss to add them both together, *"Vis unita forior"*. Joyn'd strength is strongest.

If her courses come not away as they should do, leave out the plantane, and instead thereof put mother of time.

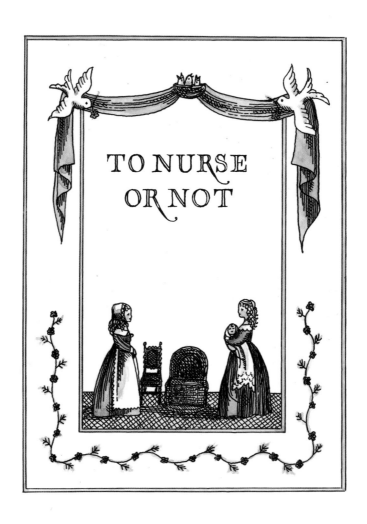

TO NURSE
OR NOT

Of nursing children.
  Oh! what a raket do authors make about this, what thwarting and contradicting, not of others only, but of themselves. What reasons do they bring why a woman must needs nurse her own child? Some extorted from divinity. Sarah nursed Isaac, thereof every woman must nurse her own child. Why is it not as good an argument, that because David was a king and a prophet, therefore everyman must be a king, and every king a prophet.

And on the other side: it would make a dying man laugh, or a horse break his halter, to hear how they thwart all this again. Say they . . . the child draws his conditions from his nurse . . . Alcibiades being an Athenian, was so strong and valiant because he sucked a Spartan woman. Cornelius Tertius strained all the wits to find out the reason, why the Germans are such strong boned men: and the result of his weak and tired brains was, because they had sucked their own mother. And why had not Alcibiades bin so if he had sucked his.

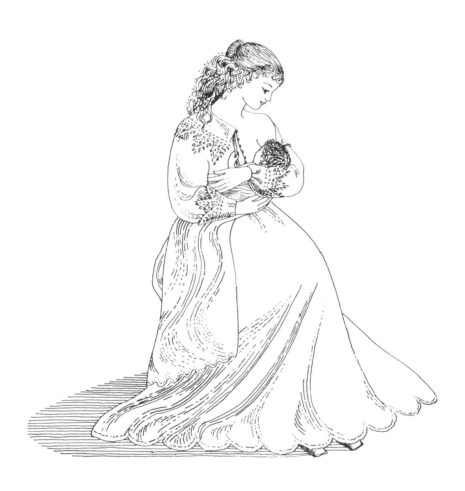

Whether an infant be better nourished by a mother or by a nurse?

Some say by a nurse; some say, the mother's milk is more like the nourishment it had in the womb which is best, except she have a disease. For he that gave her strength to conceive, travel and bring forth, will give her strength to play the nurse, though she may be weak. And honest women will be very obedient to directions, for the good of the child they love so dearly.

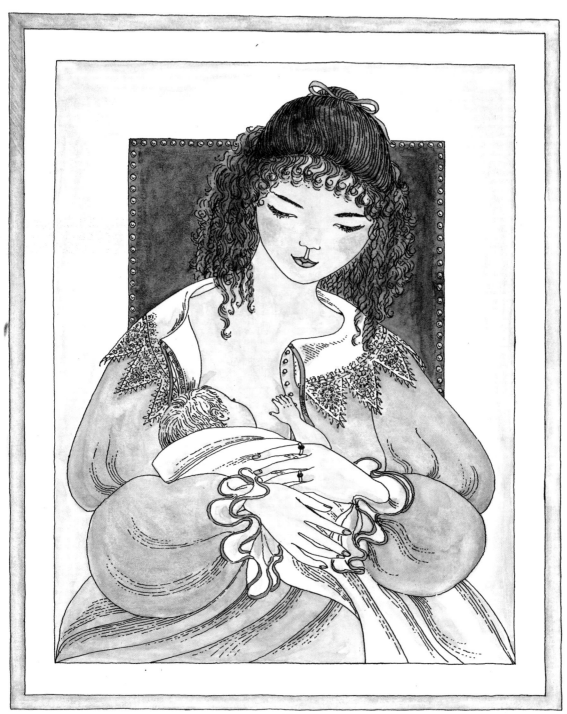

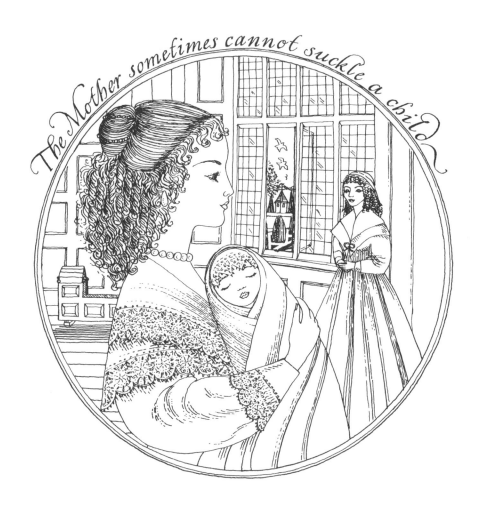

The Mother sometimes cannot suckle a child

. . . And because from weakness the mother sometimes cannot suckle a child, she must have a nurse of good habit of body, and red complexion which is the sign of the best temper, and let her not differ much from the temper; of the mother, unless it be for the better: let her be between twenty and thirty, well bred, and peaceable, not angry, melancholy, or foolish, not lecherous nor a drunkard . . . Let her breasts be well fashioned with good nipples, that the child may take to them with pleasure.

Let her keep a good diet, and abstain from hard wine and copulation, and passions: these chiefly trouble the milk.

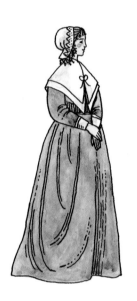

*Let her be well bred, and by it the child ... for ill bred nurses corrupt good nature. *Let her be in good health, for her own sickness infects her milk, and will be carefull of the child. *If it be a boy, let her be such a one whose last child was a boy; if a girl, contrary. *Let her be a prudent woman. *Let her nurse be such a one whose last child was a boy; let her not be with child, for she may spoil her own, or yours, or both. *Let her nurse herself, for she may spoil her own, or yours, or both. To such a nurse you may put your child.

93

?

A NURSE

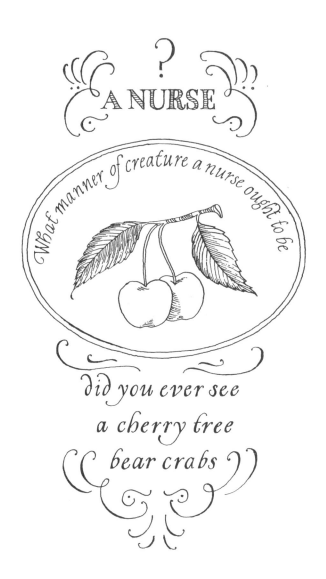

What manner of creature a nurse ought to be

did you ever see
a cherry tree
bear crabs

What manner of creature a nurse ought to be. If her complexion be fitting to make a nurse, must not her milk be good: did you ever see a cherry tree bear crabs.

I advise every good woman to choose a nurse that is a sanguine woman, and my reason is because all children in their minority have that complexion predominant.

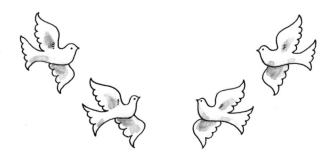

She is of middle stature, fleshy, but not fat; of a merry pleasant cheerful countenance, a ruddy color, very clear skin that you may see her veins through it.

She loves company, cannot endure to be alone; not given to anger, but infinitely to playing and singing; she delights much in children, and therefore is the fittest nurse for one.

Let her not be too poor, for if she wants, so must the child.

For age, let her be between twenty and forty for then she is in her prime.

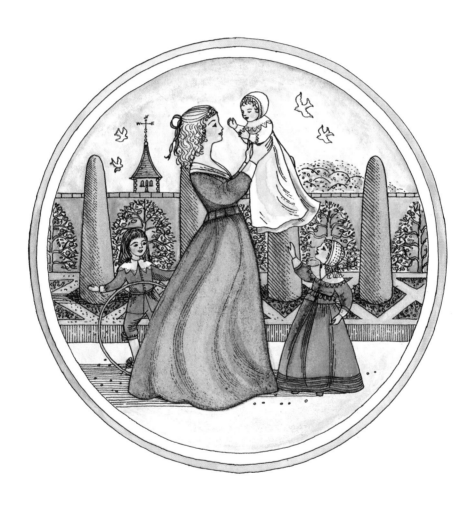

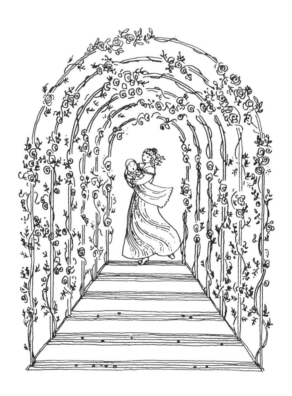

Let her use her body to exercise; if she have nothing else to do, let her dance the child.

Exercise causeth good digestion, good digestion, good blood, good blood, good milk, good milk, a thriving child.

Let her never deny herself sleep when she is sleepy, for then she will quickly awake when the child cries.

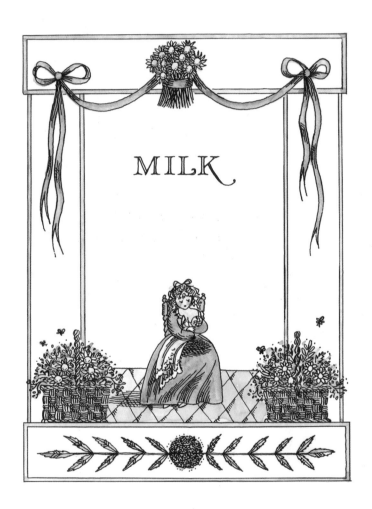

MILK

Milk digests soon, it being concocted by the nurse, and that's the reason, many in a consumption (whose digestion is weak) are cured by sucking a woman's breast.

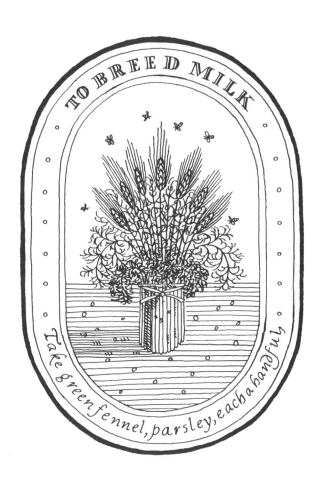

TO BREED MILK

Take green fennel, parsley, each a handful.

To breed milk, give things that breed much and good blood, of easie concoction. Medecines to breed milk, are all fennel roots, and all greens . . . These increase milk, roots of smallage, seeds of parsley, dill, basil, anise, rocket.

Compounds are: take green fennel, parsley, each a handful; barley two pugils, red prease half an ounce: boyl them and with sugar sweeten them or in chicken broath. Or,

Take green fennel six drams, barley two pugils, boil them in broath, and strain them. Or, Take fennel seed six drams, anise a dram and a half, rocket seed half a dram: give a dram or two in broath.

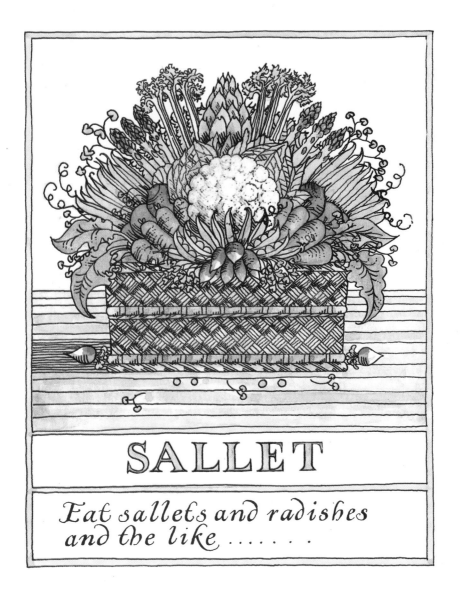

SALLET

Eat sallets and radishes and the like . . . .

There are two divers tastes, scents and colours in milk from variety of dyet. Therefore let a nurse take heed of fryed onions, and all sour, salt and spiced meats; and let her eat sallets and radishes and the like. Let her not be passionate. Milk also is sometimes salt, sharp, cholerick, and melancholick.

Correct the bloud, and keep a good diet, beware of things that corrupt the milk, as sharp, salt things; avoid anger, and other passions, and venery. Good wine moderately taken by such as have used it, takes away the ill scent from milk. If these will not do, purge the cacochymy and evil juices.

She ought to avoid all salt meats, garlick, leeks, onions and mustard. Excessive drinking of wine, strong beer or ale; for they trouble the child's body with choler. Cheese, both old and new, with melancholy: and all fish with flegm.

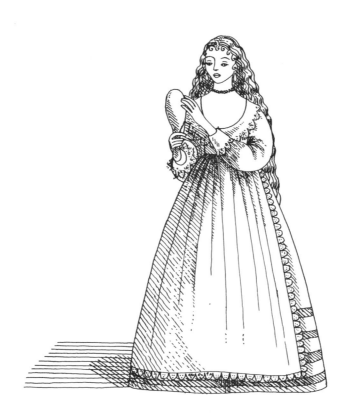

Let her shun disquietness of mind, anger, vexing and grief: for if a woman did but see her own face in a glass when she is in such passions, she would hire a man to throw stones at it.

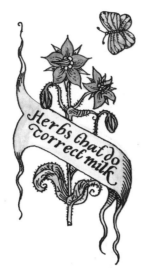

Herbs that do correct milk are these, if it be too hot, endive, and succory, lettice, sorrel, puslane and plantane. If too cold, borage, bugloss, vervain, mother of time, cinnamon, and to be brief, whatever strengthens the child in the womb, amends the milk after the woman is delivered. That thistle which is commmonly called Our Ladies thistle, because the papists thought good to dedicate it to the Blessed Virgin, whether out of a fond conceit that she amended her milk by it, I know not, yet this I know, few things growing, breed more and better milk in nurses, than that doth, and that is.

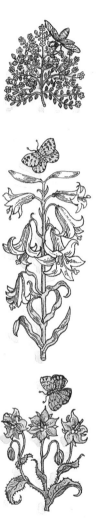
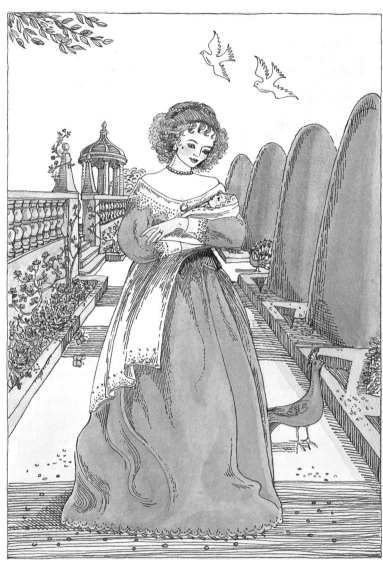
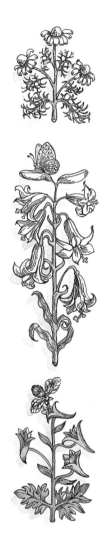

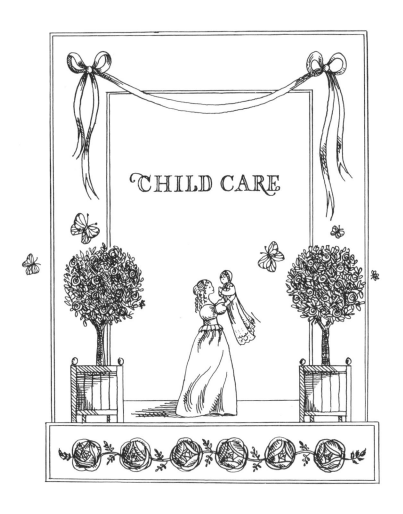

CHILD CARE

Keep it from cold air and not too hot . . . Let it not be frighted, not left alone sleeping or waking lest it receive hurt. Let it sleep long, carried in the arms often and give it the dug, but fill not too much his stomach with milk . . . Let it be often cleaned from the excrements of the belly and bladder lest they cause itching or pain or excoriation . . . A little crying empties the brain and enlargeth the lungs.

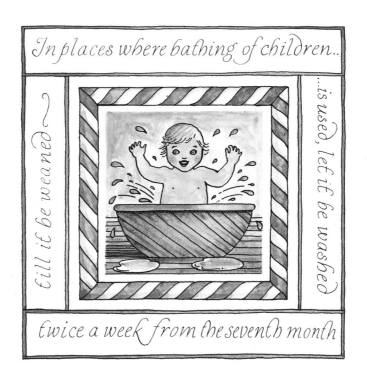

In places where bathing of children..

...is used, let it be washed

till it be weaned ∽

twice a week from the seventh month

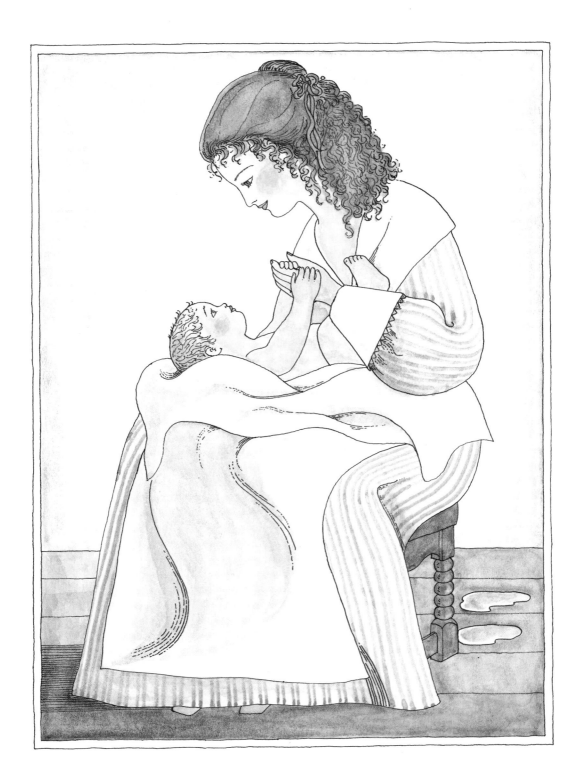

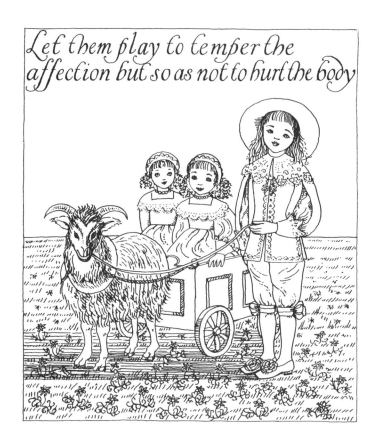

Let them play to temper the affection but so as not to hurt the body

114

For seven years the diet must be such as nourishes and causeth growth, for Hippocrates saith *"they cannot endure to fast, especially if they be witty"*. Keep them from passions, sorrow and fear and cocker them not, but keep them to reason. Let them play to temper the affection but so as not to hurt the body.

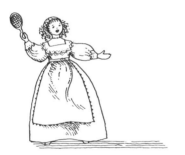

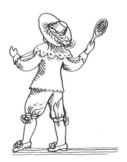

The operation of air to the body of man, is as great as meat and drink. For it helpeth to engender the vital and animal spirit, which causeth in a man, apprehension, imagination, fancy, opinion, consent, judgement, reason, resolution, discerning, knowledge, remembrance calling to mind, mirth, joy, hope, trusts, humanity, boldness, mercy, fear, sadness, dispair, hatred, malice, mildness, stubbornness, and indeed though the bulk of the body be nourished by food, the air carries the greatest swing in all the actions thereof; for it's the causer of life, health, sickness, death to mortals.

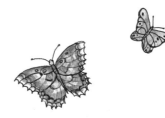

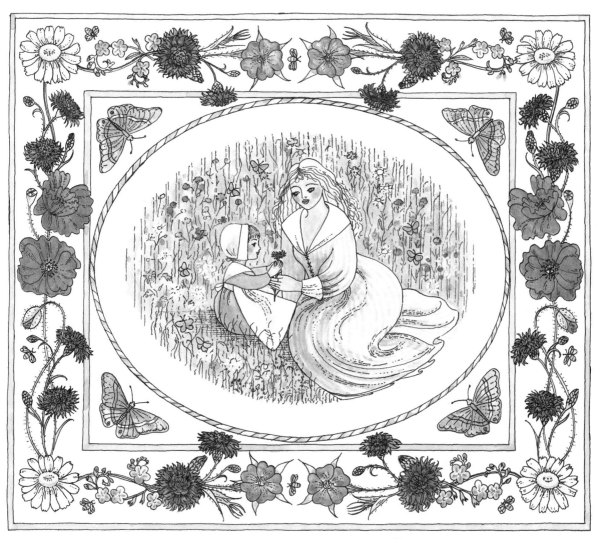

The operation of air to the body of man,
is as great as meat and drink

117

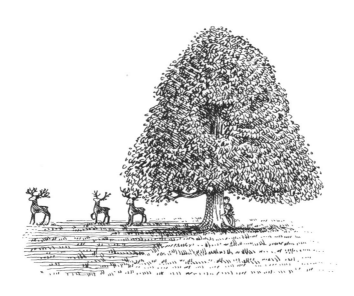

Let the air she (the nurse) lives in be good. Want of this is the reason so few children live in London, and those few that live are none the wisest, gross and thick air makes

1 Fat unwieldy bodies.
2 Dull wits.

An air near the Fens or near the sea, makes sickly bodies. Pure and clear air makes

1 Nimble bodies.
2 Quick wits.

The breathing in of ill air, and the eating of ill diet is the cause of most infirmities.

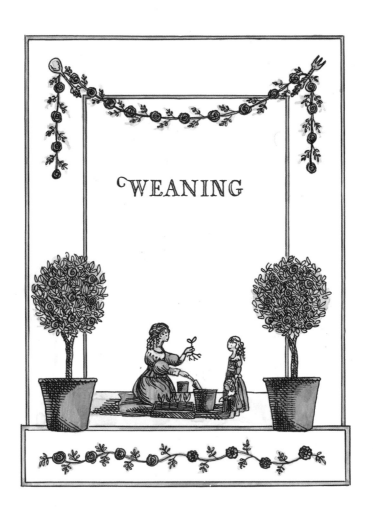

WEANING

Divide all the women in London into twenty parts, and you shall not find one of the twenty fit to be a nurse to her own child, and that for these reasons.

1 Because they give them suck too long.

2 Because they cocker them in their youth.

And that's the reason why in time, some mothers are forced to curse their children for stubbornness and ill conditions.

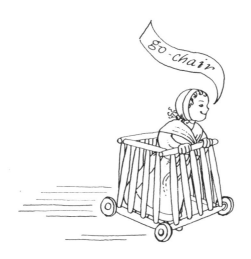

If the child be strong and healthy, a year is enough in all conscience for it to suck. Suck being ordained no longer, than until they can digest other food. The fondness of mothers to children doth them more mischief than the devil . . . in letting them suck too long. Unnatural food in their infancy, and cockering in their youth, will (if it were possible) make a devil of a saint.

When the teeth come forth, by degrees give it more solid food, and deny it not milk, such as are easily chewed. When it is stronger, let it not stand too soon, but be held by the nurse, or put into a go-chair, that it may thrust forward itself, and not fall.

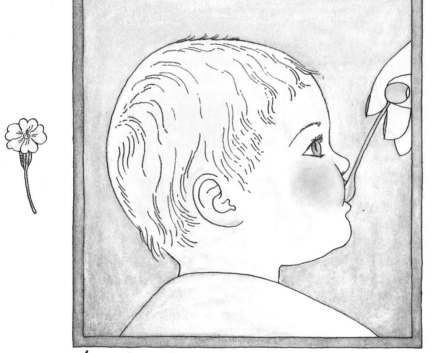

It is best to wean in the Spring and Fall,
in the increase of the moon...

Wean it not until the teeth are bred, least when the eye-teeth come forth, it cause feavers, and ache of gums and other symptoms.

The strong children must be sooner weaned than the weak, some in the twelfth, some in the fifteenth month. It is good to wean them at a year and half, or two years old, but give it not suddenly strange food, but bring it to it by degrees while it sucks.

It is best to wean in the Spring and Fall, in the increase of the moon and give but very little wine.

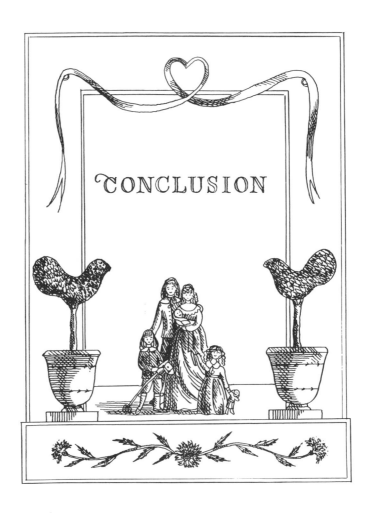

CONCLUSION

G ood women, I have for your good and not for my own, traced the beginnings of myself and you from the tools whereby we were made, and the manner we were made of, to what we were, when we were but an embryo. I have instructed you in its nourishment and growth in the womb. I have given you helps for the preservation of it there. I have given you helps to ease you in the delivery of it. I have given you orders for your body after delivery. My care hath not been wanting for the child during the time it sucks. I have not been wanting for you, freely to impart all the cautions I knew. If envy oppose me, I know that I have done well.

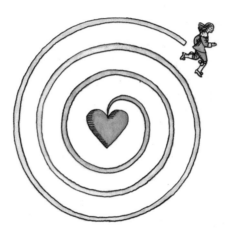

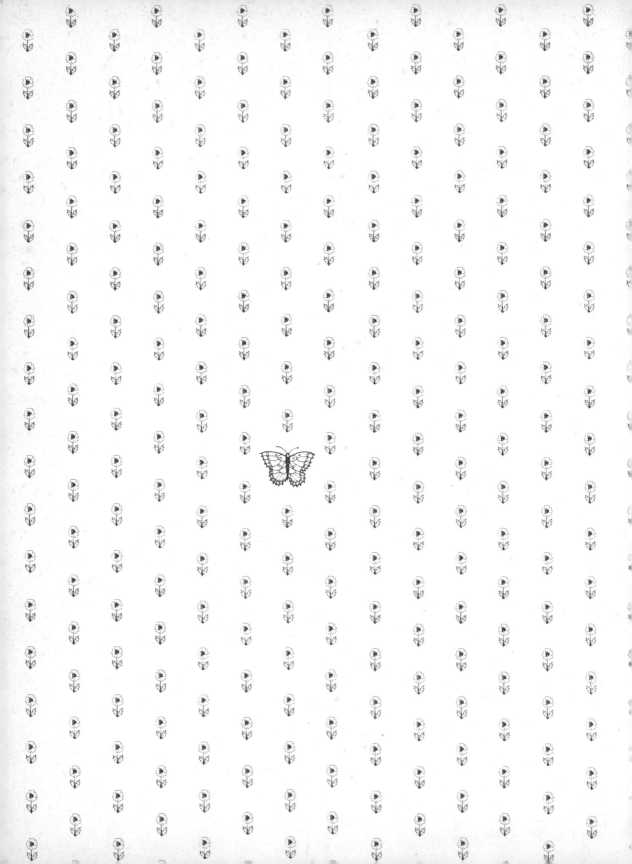